From
Health Care
To
Healthy

A Path To Regaining Health

Kurt Winowich

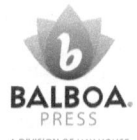

BALBOA
PRESS

A DIVISION OF HAY HOUSE

Balboa Press books may be ordered through booksellers or by contacting:

Balboa Press
A Division of Hay House
1663 Liberty Drive
Bloomington, IN 47403
www.balboapress.com
1 (877) 407-4847

Print information available on the last page.

ISBN: 978-1-4525-9798-0 (sc)
ISBN: 978-1-4525-9799-7 (e)

Library of Congress Control Number: 2014919317

Balboa Press rev. date: 01/23/2017

To my dear mother Rosemary Winowich,
who is in the process of regaining her health.
Love you Mom

Contents

Introduction ix

Chapter 1: A Spiral Downward 1
Chapter 2: Doctor Number Two 7
Chapter 3: Doctor Number Three 9
Chapter 4: Doctors Number Four and Five 13
Chapter 5: The Cruise 17
Chapter 6: Testing Your pH and Taking
            Responsibility 21
Chapter 7: Is It that Bad to Be Acidic? 27
Chapter 8: So Then What Should We Do
            to Be Healthy? 35
Chapter 9: A Spiral Upward—Addressing
            the Big Three 39
Chapter 10: Changing Your Thoughts, Changing
            Your Life 61
Chapter 11: Go for Your Dreams 65

Introduction

Our health is the single most important asset we have. The intention of this short but powerful book is to share my story of how I was able to turn around a serious health condition. The information in this book will provide you with knowledge and specifics so that you or someone you love may also have excellent health.

Chapter 1

A Spiral Downward

$\mathcal{I}$n early 2009, I developed severe gastrointestinal issues, which eventually included ulcers and borderline cancerous esophageal issues. There were many fancy names for the multiple gastrointestinal conditions I had, but the effects were simply that I could not eat any type of food without suffering severe pain for several hours after eating. Soon after the pain began to subside, it was mealtime or I would be naturally hungry, so the process would start all over again. In 2009 this condition occurred fairly infrequently, but by end of the year, my overall quality of life with my two kids, Lindsay and Christopher, my work, and my mental state were deteriorating. The following year, conditions became even worse. Every day I needed to plan where I would be so people could not see the pain I was in. Luckily I was able to work at home much of the year. When I did have to go see clients, I made the time as short as possible. I remember telling a coworker on the phone one day, "I think I'm dying." I remember lying curled up on the floor of my office after falling out of my chair. I was thinking, *I've never been shot in the stomach, but it can't hurt more than this.*

Food: What Can I Eat?

I'm about five feet eleven and 175 pounds, and if you saw me, you would likely think I look healthy. I ate pretty well, I thought. In 2009 and 2010, I experimented with foods by dropping things I was eating one by one in the hope of identifying a perpetrator. I then added new types of foods one by one with no change. I followed a list of foods that my doctor gave me, but that did not change anything. I was already doing better than what the list asked for, and I was getting more into organic foods as well. Nothing helped. In fact, it was getting slightly worse with each passing week. I was forty-nine years old and thought I might not make it to fifty.

Where Are the Doctors?

By now you're probably asking, "Is this guy just going to crumple up and cry some more, or is he going to get to a doctor already? Sheesh!" Let's back up a bit. In 2008- 2009, I had lower-back problems from injuries I had sustained in my twenties. Stress has a way of finding a weak point in your body and then exploiting it. I had gone to my doctor, whom I trusted and felt a connection with. He prescribed a painkiller and anti-inflammatory to be used as needed. Well, I needed it all the time, so I used it all the time and became addicted. My lower back did not get better, but my stomach began to hurt. My doctor suggested some exercises, but painkillers make you want to do less, not more. If you've ever taken painkillers or narcotics, you will notice one of the first things that happens is you become constipated. In my case, I remember going from success in the bathroom to nothing happening for a week at a time. Now, it doesn't take a genius to realize that if you are eating and taking drugs but not eliminating, all of those toxins remain in your system and begin to break down otherwise healthy tissue in your body. Keep in mind that even after finally having a bowel movement seven days later, we remain backed up as long as we continue taking the drug. This keeps more toxins and acid in the body, which creates further breakdowns in tissue. The drug companies call these *side effects*.

As time passes, an increase in dosage is required to get the same effect that it had before. So as you increase the dosage to bear the pain, you are also constipating yourself further, and your body becomes toxic rather quickly. Many prescription drugs have this effect. Suddenly, you're in a downward spiral. My doctor failed to mention any of these hazards to me, and since I trusted him, I failed to read every line of the attached documentation or go to the website for further information. It's kind of like buying a car: we don't sit and read every line in the contract as we are purchasing. We trust that what we are buying isn't going to kill us but will make us happy we came in. That may be because if we actually read the information about the particular drug and researched it, the logical choice would be to not take it. When you are in severe pain, however, you just want the pain to stop as soon as possible. My doctor also prescribed a well-known sleep medication because the pain was preventing me from sleeping. The sleep medication worked at first but then tapered off until it really did nothing to promote sleep. If I didn't take it for one night, however, I would not be able to sleep at all.

As we rolled into 2010, my stomach and whole digestive tract was beginning to hurt, and I began to have acid burning all the way up to my throat. I ate Tums and drank bottles of Pepto-Bismol for weeks with no relief before again heading back to my doctor. This time I came limping in with back pain like the first time but now with some additional problems. My back still hurt because I wasn't solving the issue; I was attempting to cover up the pain that was still there. Now I was severely constipated with pains from the top of my stomach up to my heart. I had never had heartburn before, but I thought, *Well, lots of people get heartburn. I'll be okay.* My doctor looked at me and did the normal nodding and prodding, checking and poking. He then prescribed me a very well-known acid-reflux drug. He said, "You have acid-reflux disease, my man."

I said, "Disease? How did I suddenly develop a disease?"

He said, "Well, lots of people get this. It probably won't kill you, but we're going to send you in for an endoscopy."

I asked, "How long after the endoscopy will I need to take this drug?"

He said, "Forever!"

This drug basically suppresses the production of acid in your gastrointestinal area, so I started taking it. I did the endoscopy. They put a small camera down your esophagus and look around. I visited my doctor to review the results.

There were a couple of ulcers and burns on the wall of my esophagus, and while this was obviously not good, my doctor said he didn't think I should have the amount of stomach pain I had, and he referred me to a well-known gastrointestinal specialist.

Chapter 2

Doctor Number Two

*B*y the time I got in to see the gastrointestinal doctor, six weeks had passed due to his eternally full schedule. *Why do so many people have gastro problems?* I thought. So I limped in, my back and stomach severely hurting. I was now taking three drugs, and when I saw the second doctor—the gastrointestinal specialist—I was in worse shape than when I had started a couple months earlier.

The physician's assistant ordered some tests and imaging to look around inside. Maybe she thought I had swallowed an anvil or something. It sure felt like it! We did an ultrasound, a CAT scan, and an X-ray of my stomach area. Before I went to schedule my tests, she prescribed a stomach tranquilizer for my pain. She said it should calm things down in my stomach. After I scheduled my imaging tests, I picked up the new medicine and began taking it twice a day. The drug did calm down my body—so much so that I had trouble seeing my computer screen to do my work. It blurred my vision and made me just want to lie down. That would have been fine, but I had two kids to raise as a single father, a house to take care of, and a career. The pain was still there, and I was still curling up on the floor to the point of tears sometimes.

After meeting with the physician's assistant, I went to see a spine doctor, who diagnosed me with scoliosis and a severely stuck sacroiliac joint. He recommended surgery, as surgeons do. Surgery, however, didn't feel like the right answer—at least not yet. I found a couple of different chiropractors, and they both seemed to make the condition worse. Looking back, I believe we didn't spend enough time analyzing my condition before proceeding. I stopped seeing them and refocused on getting a cure to my gastrointestinal pains. I did have the knowledge of my diagnosis, however, which I planned to do my own research on.

I was now taking four very powerful drugs: the pain drug for my back, the sleeping pill, the antacid, and the stomach tranquilizer. It's not hard to imagine that with all the side effects of these drugs, I was feeling worse, but with the upcoming tests, I felt hopeful we would get to the bottom of this with the expertise of a gastrointestinal specialist. It took a couple of weeks to complete the first two imaging exams and then a couple more weeks for the third exam.

Once the results came back, my gastrointestinal specialist called me in to review it. We sat down, and I got a bit excited about figuring this out and getting me well again. As she looked over the charts and images, she said, "Mr. Winowich, I have some good news and bad news. The good news is we found nothing wrong with you—no blockages, etc. The bad news is we found nothing wrong with you."

Chapter 3

Doctor Number Three

$\mathscr{S}$ince weeks and months had gone by with no improvement, I decided I needed to see the most senior gastro doctor in the establishment. I asked to have an appointment with this doctor, and the staff acted as if I was asking to see God himself. The waiting list was long. I secured an appointment with the senior gastro doctor, and while I was waiting, I was scheduled to take another battery of tests that the gastro specialist ordered. These included blood work for celiac disease, urine porphyries, ESR, and CRP. There was also one more imaging exam that was very uncomfortable called a HIDA exam.

As bad as I felt leaving still with no answers and hurting terribly, I was hopeful we were on the right track by working through tests and moving up on the doctor food chain. I was determined to get this figured out by process of elimination if needed. I went through the lab tests and the HIDA exam. During the HIDA exam, my back was hurting so bad they had to put pillows under my left leg to keep me still long enough to complete the exam. I had now taken about every imaging test and upper GI test known, short of a colonoscopy. As bad as I felt because of the stomach pain, I was still hopeful that these tests would show something my new gastro doctor would be able to identify so we could fix it and I could get back to life.

As I progressed through 2010, my corporate job really began to see how ill I was. I didn't go into the office much so as to not draw too much attention. I was still able to do my design work at the computer and make phone calls. I did most of my work from my home office, which I appreciated. What people could not see over the phone was that I was hunched over when I walked due to pain in my stomach and back. All of the meds made me so I was unable to genuinely smile. I wasn't happy and felt like an angry dog sometimes. It felt like I was just in survival mode, and I did not want my managers at the office to see me this way. Everyone at the office was great, however within two hours of eating anything, the pain would get so bad every day that I would have to lie down and curl up, which I could not do at the office.

One day, as I was coming home from making an appearance at the office, the pain became unusually bad. I was driving and thought, *I'm not going to make it home. I can't focus on the road.* I drove straight to the hospital here in Clearwater, Florida. I practically crawled into the emergency room doors. A man brought me a wheelchair since he saw I could barely walk. I checked into the emergency room and then stayed in the wheelchair and waited. After sitting for about two hours in extreme pain, I rolled back to the desk and mentioned, "I can't sit here much longer like this.

I'm beginning to lose my mind over the pain." *People with stomachaches obviously don't get priority,* I thought.

I sat there for another hour before they rolled me back to check me out. I remember thinking, *Maybe here there will be a doctor who can figure out what is wrong with me. Please, please, please, please—there has to be someone here who can* fix *me!* After all of the questions and answers they documented, a nurse put me in a bed to wait for a doctor. For the next two hours, someone would occasionally open the curtain and walk in. Each time I got excited, only to then see that it was just someone to check my blood pressure again or adjust my pillow or something else I felt was unimportant.

I kept asking, "When is a doctor going to come?"

The answer was always, "Soon."

"I've been here for five hours in severe pain and just want to see a doctor. Please, I'm in pain," I said.

My emotions and my attitude were being affected by all the meds I was taking, plus the stress of the pain. At one point there were three nurses in my room trying to calm me down as I squirmed around on the bed. I felt like the guy on the table in the movie *Alien,* and I really thought maybe there was something inside me that was going to suddenly make an appearance. After two more hours of being told the doctor would be there soon, I realized I could not take it anymore, so I got up and started to walk out.

As soon as I started to leave, the nurse said, "Wait, you can't just walk out. The doctor is coming."

I thought about the thousands of dollars in medical insurance I paid and I had to sit there for seven hours in pain. I would have rather been home, so I left while the nurse followed me for a bit, trying to get me to come back to sign some more papers, which I did not. I went home and curled up on the bed until the pain subsided. Do you know the hospital still sent me a bill for hundreds of dollars even though they never sent a doctor to see me?

My appointment with my new gastro doctor finally arrived. I had hoped that this top-notch, highly qualified, experienced doctor would surely be able to mull over all of the details and finally figure out what was wrong in my body. When I met with this doctor, we reviewed all of the drugs I was on, and then he proceeded to explain that all of the tests had come back negative. The blood work, the urine test, the ESR and CRP, and the HIDA exam all came back negative. He then claimed there were no more tests that he knew of that could help identify the problem. He explained that I had irritable bowel syndrome, acid reflux disease, and ulcers.

"Wow," I said. "A syndrome and a disease—now we're getting somewhere. So what is the cure for these?"

I was actually excited that we had identified the issues and now we could solve them. After all, that is what I do all day long as a technology architect—I solve problems, and I know there is a solution to every problem. The doctor then gave me his answer.

He said, "Well, since we don't know what causes these issues, we don't really have a cure. It's a matter of finding the right medicine to alleviate the symptoms."

That was then when I realized this doctor was not looking for a cause but only wanted to address the symptoms with drugs. I left this doctor's office and decided I needed to find the right doctor—that was all.

Chapter 4

Doctors Number Four and Five

I took my prognosis, looked for the most famous gastro doctor I could find in Tampa, and set an appointment. I rounded up all of my images, test results, and drugs I'd been taking and went to see a gastro expert in Tampa. As I was sitting in the new doctor's waiting room, I noticed all of the doctor's degrees in medicine and the associations he belonged to. They were very impressive. I was again hopeful that we could solve these painful conditions I had. You see, I refused to label the conditions I had as a disease or syndrome. I believe doctors use these terms to help you succumb and realize there is no cure, all of which promotes fear, thereby causing people to get with the program and do what the doctor says.

What I liked about this new doctor (even though I had not seen him yet) was that he asked for all of my records, images, and test results two weeks ahead of time so he would know what my issues were when I walked in. They called me into the room, and the doctor came in and said, "Sounds like you're in some pain?"

"Every day," I said.

The doctor began to explain that he had gone over everything and it sounded like the other doctors were on the right track. I told him, "I am having trouble with all of the drugs I'm taking. They make me tired. I can't seem to focus on anything, and I don't take them every day because they turn me into a zombie and don't seem to help."

The doctor then proceeded to explain that what he saw in the images showed that my disease could become cancerous and that I needed to take the drugs every day to control the acid. I said, "So is it the acid that is causing all of my troubles?"

He said, "I believe it is one of the main factors."

I asked, "Where is the acid coming from?"

He said, "From you. Your body is producing too much acid."

I then said, "Why is my body producing too much acid?"

He said, "It's hard to say. A lot of people have this condition. The point is we need to control the acid, and the drugs are how we do that."

"So how long will I have to take the drugs?"

"Forever," he said. "There are some new medicines out that may work better for you."

He wrote me a script, and I left after making another appointment to report back on the new meds. On the way home, I thought we had gotten closer to the cause of my issue, but I refused to believe my stomach was the cause of my issues and that the answer was more drugs. I could see that this doctor was going to give me more of the same, so I decided to look for yet another doctor.

One night I received a call from a manager of the company I worked for. He told me our global corporation had a service that helped to find the best doctor for a given condition. I decided I needed to take advantage of this service. Again collecting all of my records, I was hopeful that I would find the doctor who could fix me. About thirty days after submitting all of my records, an expert gastro doctor out of Boston sent me a report based on all of my records. There was no reason to see me in person, they said. The report basically named a couple different drugs to try and that I might be allergic to wheat products. I wasn't eating wheat products. They summed it up by saying it sounded like a case of irritable bowel syndrome.

This is basically the name of a condition that they do not know the cause of or the cure for. Many gastro conditions are labeled IBS, which means the doctors will provide drugs for it but have no idea how to cure it. I had been to four doctors, even expert doctors who only dealt with gastrointestinal issues, and in the end, they couldn't help me. The pain was terrible, and mentally I needed an attitude adjustment.

I had been through the best health care system on planet earth, and two years later I was no better. I began to think sometimes that this thing was going to kill me if I didn't solve it.

> People need to realize they are not ill due to
> a lack of pharmaceutical drugs in the body.
> —K. T.

Chapter 5

The Cruise

*F*or twenty plus years, I've been an avid reader of self-development books and courses. One day I was exposed to a success club—a brand-new club that claimed to help people be, do, or have whatever they wanted. I knew that if I kept focusing on this illness, it wasn't going to go away. I realized I needed to think about something else to get my attention off of being ill. I signed up and joined this club to begin to obtain information via a website and later meetings that would help people reach their goals.

The club announced there would be a cruise in January 2011, which was two months away. I thought, *Gosh, that sounds fun, but I feel so bad. There is no way I can go.* I was doing very little those days, staying close to home and away from people and too much excitement. Something kept telling me, though, that I *had* to be on this cruise. My brain kept saying, "A cruise is the last thing you want to do right now, Kurt." But my feelings were telling me I had to go, so I signed up for the cruise, got a new passport, and waited for January.

A week before the cruise, I was hurting so bad that I told my kids, "I just can't go."

My eighteen-year-old daughter said, "Dad, you have to go." It was probably so she could have a party while I was gone, but in either case, she was right. It made no logical sense that I would go on this self-development cruise being as ill as I was, but I knew I had to go.

Once on the ship, I began to meet and make friends with people from all over the world with as many backgrounds— from CIA agents to ex-congressmen to natural healers of the mind and body. After reading the session schedules, I decided that the first session I would attend was one put on by a guy named Ted Morter of Morter Health Systems. Ted is the son of Milton Morter, creator of the BEST system—bio energetic synchronization technique. He was a true pioneer in health care of the mind and body. I had never heard of or seen anything like what I saw in the session. I watched someone right before my eyes be healed of a fairly serious physical ailment. The person on the receiving end is a good friend of mine now almost four years later, and although at the time I thought there may have been some trickery involved, I now know there was not. Could it actually be true that someone with serious health conditions who had not been able to heal could actually get well in a matter of minutes in some cases? It was really hard to believe, and in fact at the time on the ship I really couldn't believe it and thought, *They are trying to sell something here.*

After the session I knew I had to at least say hi to Dr. Ted Morter but Dr. Ted had so many people around him. I was in pain as usual and decided I would try to say hello to him later if I ran into him on the ship again. As I turned to leave the room, I locked eyes with an older gentleman who was sitting in the front row. He had been watching me I think, and I said, "I wanted to ask Dr. Ted about my stomach," as I was holding one hand over my stomach.

The older gentleman said, "What's wrong with your stomach?"

I said, "It always hurts. I can't eat right, and my digestive tract is destroyed."

The older gentleman then asked me something that changed my entire life. He asked, "What is your pH?"

"My pH?" I said. "I have no idea. No doctor has ever asked me that before."

The older gentleman just nodded and said, "Find out."

I then nodded, and as the room became noisier, I walked out. A little later a friend who I met earlier saw me and asked what I was talking to Dr. Morter about. I said, "Oh, I didn't get to speak with Dr. Morter."

My friend said, "I saw you chatting with Dr. Morter Sr."

"Oh, was that Dr. Milton Morter?" I asked.

My friend said, "Yes."

Now I knew I had chatted with the developer of Morter Health Systems, and I wrote down what he said to do—check my pH.

Throughout the remainder of the cruise, I met and chatted with some very successful authors—people like John Gray, author of *Men Are from Mars, Women Are from Venus*," Mary Miller, creator of I-ching Systems, and Kevin Trudeau, who is extremely knowledgeable in so many areas and a health expert himself. What I later discovered was that these people as well as most people on the cruise were there to not only talk and learn about success principles but also about how important good health is. These speakers were not just authors or speakers; they were experts in health, promoting true health. Health was always at the top of the agendas of these highly successful people.

I was given a list of books to read before I left the cruise, so upon leaving for home I had my notes and a list of books to find and begin reading. When I got home and read the list of recommended reading, I was surprised to find that not one of the books was on health. These incredible books were on topics such as believing and thinking and feeling emotions, dreaming, and visualization. *Why no books on health?* I thought.

What I later discovered after reading these and other books is that good health as well as illness both begin in the mind. Get your thinking right, or your mind right, and you will then do the things necessary for your well-being. You see, negative thinking or worse, negative feelings bring on conditions for illness. On the other hand, a positive attitude or always "looking for the gold," as my mentor would say, creates conditions for a healthy body and mind. We will discuss this more in the last chapter, but for now, just know that mental clarity and mental health are prerequisites to physical health. Emotional stress and negative thinking wear down the immune system and places hardship on every cell in your body, opening you up for illness.

Chapter 6

Testing Your pH and Taking Responsibility

*F*ollowing the five seconds of advice I received from Dr. Milton Morter on the cruise, I decided to circle back with my original family doctor. This was the doctor who recommended I see the gastro doctors two years earlier. I went in and decided to tell him what I had learned and asked him about pH.

When I met the doctor, I said, "Look, Doctor, I really want to stop taking all of these drugs. I met some other doctors that told me drugs are toxic to the body, and by the way, what is my pH?"

Then the doctor said something that made me realize I would never see him again after almost ten years of being in his care. He said, "Well, I'm a medical doctor, and we've not tested your pH. If you stop taking two of the drugs, you could have some serious trouble, including cancer." His point was, "I'm a medical doctor, and if you don't want to take drugs, there is nothing I can do for you." He finally said, "Rather than a blood test, you should be able to test your pH yourself." So I left to go find pH test strips. He said any pharmacy or drug store would have them.

As I went in search of pH strips, it came over me suddenly that I had just made the decision to fire my doctor and take 100 percent responsibility for solving my health issues and getting healthy. I decided I was going to learn for myself about the mind and body and do whatever it takes to get myself healthy, with or without a medical doctor. The few seconds I spent with Dr. Morter had a compelling impact on me, and I had to find out what my pH level was. I was going to do whatever research I needed to do in order to get myself healthy. I had waited for two years for some answers from all of my doctors and was given none. I was going to find the answers, and I suddenly became empowered.

I hit all the major pharmacies and drug stores in search of pH test strips. To my surprise, none of these stores sold the test strips. When I asked why, the pharmacist just said, "We don't carry them anymore."

One pharmacist, with a puzzled look on his face, said, "Why do you want to know your pH?"

I said, "Because someone told me it's important."

The pharmacist said, "You can probably find test strips at a garden center where people test the soil for pH balance."

Later I learned that all drugs, be they illegal, pharmaceutical, or over the counter, (even aspirin) cause acidity in the body. A body that is acidic as opposed to pH balanced allows illness and disease to flourish. So the very thing that the pharmacy was selling (drugs) actually caused a pH to be imbalanced or acidic. I didn't realize it at the time, but now I no longer wonder why you won't find pH test strips at the pharmacy, at least no where I live in Clearwater, Florida.

Somehow putting a soil test strip in my mouth didn't sound like a good idea, although now I know that is perfectly fine and works. Rather I simply went online to eBay and found a medical product supplier and purchased a whole lot for a few bucks. The test strips came in the mail a few days later. They have a small, easy-to-read color chart included so you can easily read the numbers after you expose the strip to saliva or urine.

While I was waiting for the strips to arrive, I did some research on pH and found Dr. Morter online talking about the importance of balanced pH for health and well-being and how pH is an indicator of health and can be changed if needed. As I did more research, I found that back in the 1930s in Nazi Germany, there was a doctor and scientist named Heinrich Warburg. Warburg won a Nobel Prize for his work during that time. What Warburg discovered and documented was how cancer cells flourish in an acidic environment but not in an alkaline environment. His studies showed that the cells of our bodies break down under the stress of an acidic state in the body. The Nazis kept this doctor around even though he had Jewish blood. That was how important this study was to the Nazis.

I waited until the following morning to do the pH tests. I learned that first thing in the morning is the best time to test our pH level as we have not eaten or drunk anything that could dilute the results. The next morning I took out the test strips and did a urine sample on one and a saliva sample on the other. After a minute, the colors showed clearly that I had a pH in both cases of about 6.1.

Now a pH of 6.1 may not sound bad when you consider a perfect pH balance is 7.4. My 6.1 pH reading meant, however, that I was about fifteen to thirty times more acidic than a balance of 7.4. A pH reading of 7.4 is the balance marker that indicates the right balance of alkaline and acid needed to maintain good health of our bodies. I continued to test each morning for the following week in order to get an average of my pH reading. I was as low as 6.0 and as high as 6.5, and I calculated my pH average for that timeframe at about 6.2.

Now there are some who will argue that your saliva and urine are not good indicators of your true pH level and that a blood test is the only true indicator. The blood pH level is maintained by whatever means is necessary by the body even when that means that bones and vital organs need to be robbed of certain minerals and or elements. As organs and other body systems are robbed of nutrients to maintain pH balance in the blood, those organs and systems attempt to protect themselves from breakdown but can only do so much for so long. If we aren't consuming the right things and are exposing ourselves to the wrong things, that will show up in our saliva and urine tests in an acidic pH reading. That means the body is in survival mode and attempting to protect itself using whatever means necessary, which causes other issues. My research showed that being in a long-term acidic state can lead to all major ailments and illnesses. One of the most widespread conditions caused by acidity in the body is inflammation. Inflammation around joints, organs like the heart, and other body systems is caused by the body attempting to protect itself from the acid, which breaks down cells. Inflammation acts like a buffer to basically keep you alive, but as you will see in the upcoming examples, it causes other problems that are painful and devastating in some cases.

Keep in mind as you read the following examples that later in the book we will talk about the causes of becoming acidic and how to avoid it and correct it. There are many diseases and disorders that are associated with an acidic condition, such as cataracts, arthritis, osteoporosis, gout, cancer, migraines, constipation, morning sickness, stroke, allergies, diabetes, obesity, etc.

Note that a person does not catch these conditions out of thin air. These are conditions that are developed by the individual person. You don't catch arthritis like a cold, and you aren't handed arthritis by your mother or father. A condition or disease is something that develops over time and therefore can be reversed in time. With this awareness of how acidity affects us, we can all choose to make informed and healthier decisions for wellness, which we will talk about later in the book.

Chapter 7

Is It that Bad to Be Acidic?

*T*he following are just some of the common and major body systems that are negatively affected by having an acidic state in the body and some of the conditions or diseases that come from that long-term exposure. The body has responses to acidity that basically create protective inflammation to halt sudden death. Over time, however, these protective measures create new conditions that we call degenerative diseases.

1. **Circulatory System**: Heart disease is caused by being acidic. Why? The heart has to protect itself from the acidic environment. Why? Because acid can burn right through a heart artery, and then it's game over. The well-meaning heart, in all of its wisdom, begins to protect itself from the acidic environment by creating a protective barrier inside of the arteries. This is known as fat plaque, a form of inflammation. If the acidic condition isn't corrected, the heart

will continue to put more space between the acid coming through and the artery wall by creating more inflammation. It isn't hard to figure out what eventually can happen. The artery eventually does not provide enough room for blood flow to occur easily, and the heart eventually becomes overworked (i.e., heart attack).

2. **Digestive Tract:** Digestive problems, such as gastric reflux, indigestion, nausea, and bloating, are caused by being acidic. Too much acid in the digestive tract can cause many issues, the least of which are ulcers and esophageal spasms, which is what I had. The pain can be unbearable. Most people go to the doctor and obtain powerful anti-acid drugs. These drugs can keep the acid at bay but come with a host of side effects first and foremost being that acid and enzymes, which are needed to digest food correctly, are also suppressed. When food isn't digested efficiently, you get backed up, and that creates more acid to break down the food, which requires stronger drugs to suppress. Do you see a vicious cycle here? That is why I called it a spiral downward in chapter 1.

3. **Immune System:** Being acidic wears down the immune system. Bad bacteria can flourish in the cells of our bodies when those cells are acidic. Cells that become acidic and are not pH balanced lack oxygen and proper circulation, as well as proper elimination. When germs invade the body, as they do all day long each day, cells that are acidic are weak and open to attack and to spreading those germs. A

weak immune system is therefore caused by an acidic lifestyle and an acidic condition. A strong immune system comes from having properly oxygenated cells that expel toxins efficiently and therefore are healthy, vibrant, and not susceptible to the attack of germs. When people take cold medicines of any type, they are actually making themselves more acidic. Those medicines are toxins that worsen the state of the cells further. Those medicines do nothing to help the body heal itself. They are there to really only numb out the pain or discomfort, which again is polluting the body further. Next time you have a cold or flu, drink tea, get your vitamins C and D3, rest, and drink lots of water. Help your body do what it knows how to do, heal itself.

4. **Skeletal System**: Arthritis or inflammation of the joints is developed when one is acidic in most cases. It is not developed from overworking the joints. As the lubricating fluids of the joints become acidic, the joints become dryer and begin to get irritated and swell. As more and more acid deposits itself into the joint areas, the inflammation continues to get worse and affects mobility and strength. Additional swelling also occurs as the body attempts to create a protection layer between bones and cartilage while trying to deal with the acid.

There are many more examples of just how an acidic condition creates damage to our bodily systems, including the reproductive, brain, urinary, muscular, and nervous systems. Do your own follow-up research.

"One of the single most important things you can do for your health" is to test your pH level. That is a bold statement and probably something you have never heard before. The reason many health care practitioners can say this is simple. If having an acidic pH balance is what opens you up to illness and diseases, then keeping your pH balance in check will keep you healthy.

Does that mean you will never get a cold or a cough or an ache or a pain? No, of course not, but if you do catch something, your body will have the ability to attack and subdue the minor intrusion effectively. Your body will do what it is designed to do. If we find our pH is out of balance, it is only a matter of figuring out what we are doing or not doing to create that imbalance and then correcting it. We will be talking about these things later. Our pH balance tells us if we are doing enough of the right things for our bodies or doing too many of the wrong things. Knowing what these things are may take a bit of an education, but it will be fun. Hopefully this book is the starting place for your journey of change. Feeling good is everyone's natural state. If you are feeling bad most of the time, it is only a matter of identifying those things that need to change, and it is not complicated. You just need to alkalize your body back to balance.

Before we move on to the topic of prevention and remedy, let's summarize a few things and tie some things together. First, know that most people walking around are acidic and don't know it. They don't know what they don't know and therefore are doing nothing to correct it. Doctors do not generally test your pH when you visit for ailments or checkups. Therefore people doubt that it could be that important. The answer again is if you are ill, your pH has become out of balance, and correcting that balance is how you will resolve your illness—period. How is it that we here in the mighty United States of America are always in the top five countries in the world for cancer rates? There are over 160 countries, some with over a billion people. Don't we in the United States have the best doctors, the best health care system, the best medical schools, and the most money and resources?

Why is it that the rate of heart disease, cancer, diabetes, and many other conditions are on the rise and are not being diminished here in the United States? Why aren't more people being cured? Why aren't more people able to avoid or correct these conditions when we have so many resources devoted to "fighting" these conditions? Are these fair questions? Our health care system has some of the smartest, most well-educated people on planet earth. Our health care system is called the finest health care system on planet earth, and I'm not saying that it is not. Just remember that in the end, our health care system is one of our largest businesses here in the United States, and in the end, it is made up of corporations. These corporations have a goal in mind, and that is to make money and deliver to stockholders. If I am in the restaurant business, I need hungry people, but if I am in the health care business, I need sick people. Healthy people do not help my business if my business is health care.

Our mainstream health care system is dedicated to treating the symptoms of illness and disease, not curing or preventing the causes of illness or disease. Many people know this instinctually but don't know what else to do. This is due to heavy programming by the media, our families, the belief systems we have developed, and society in general. Until you correct the cause of the condition (or imbalance), you have not cured anything. Does this make sense?

Aristotle once said, "If you prove the *cause*, you at once prove the *effect*; and conversely nothing can exist without its *cause*." Each day, we as individuals are either at cause or effect, and make no mistake, it is our personal choices that put us at one or the other. If we don't like a particular effect we are experiencing, we need to identify the cause and either eliminate it or change it. We can't go about changing the effect without changing the cause. Medical symptoms are effects of a cause or causes. Eliminate the cause and you eliminate the effect or symptoms.

This reminds me of a joke. A girl walks into the doctor's office and says, "Doctor, it hurts when I do this."

The doctor replies, "Well, don't do that."

A condition is therefore an effect of a cause, which is something we have been doing to our bodies or not doing for our bodies. We then develop conditions like heart disease, cancer, diabetes, etc. People were not born with these conditions and did not catch them from the air. The conditions were self-inflicted, unknowingly caused and created by each individual person. Although that may sound like bad news, it is actually the greatest news because it points out that the person is the cause of his or her conditions. Again, if we don't like the effects, we can identify and make changes to the causes. A symptom is merely an indicator that there is a cause out there that needs to be addressed. The longer we wait, the more impressive that symptom will become.

Your pH is an indicator of the health of your body, and if it is not in balance, we need to find the cause. If I am acidic, the question then becomes, "What am I doing or not doing that is the cause of me being acidic?" The good news is that there really are only a few basic reasons. Will all of the changes that may be required work overnight? Probably not. After all, you didn't obtain the condition overnight. However, you can start to feel better fairly quickly. Forget the notion of taking a pill to instantly resolve something and feel better. Think about getting your body back in balance, however long it takes, so you can feel good again long term.

Once I was able to see my pH balance (tested from my saliva and urine each morning) at around 7.0 fairly consistently, the pain began to go away in my gut. My ulcers healed, and my esophagus issues began to cease. The extreme acid reflux I once had wasn't gone yet, but it was significantly reduced. As time went on and I learned more about the right things to do and what not to do, the conditions diminished more and more. The pain in my back also went away as it was due mostly to inflammation.

Today I can say that I don't take any medications, even the ones the doctors told me I would have to take forever. Again, I make no medical claims here, and before you make any sudden changes such as reducing or removing drugs from your lifestyle, speak with your doctor. I am not advocating that you stop taking your medications cold turkey. There could be major side effects in doing that. I am merely sharing that I was able to taper off and completely stop taking all medications only after I brought my body into balance. I am simply sharing what I and many others have done to regain excellent health. As a matter of fact, I am fifty-three years old and recently applied for a life insurance policy with a top company here in the United States. After all of the health tests were finished, I received the highest rating possible for anyone who would like a policy with this company. I don't tell you this to impress you but to point out that if I can do it, so can you.

Chapter 8

So Then What Should We Do to Be Healthy?

isclaimer: I make no claims to be a doctor or practitioner of any kind. The information here is purely my opinion based on my experience and others' opinions, both practitioners and nonpractitioners. I claim no cures for any disease here, although the information referenced here has helped me as well as others.

- *Why it's not health care*: There are necessary drugs and surgery, but they should only be used for urgent medical care to save your life. It's great that we have drugs and surgery in these cases, of course. Drugs are toxins and are not for the care of your health or for everyday consumption. You are not ill due to a lack of pharmaceutical drugs in your body. You are ill because you are doing or not doing something to your mind and body and therefore are allowing the illness to continue.

- *My credentials:* My experience as a patient of the American healthcare system gives me my credentials. Because I spent a lot of time in pain with no results, I was motivated to discover the practitioners, technology, and resources that actually do promote health care. Again, if you are happy with the treatment you are receiving from your medical doctor, then the following information is not for you. If, however, you find that you are simply taking a drug to suppress an illness symptom and find yourself obtaining new conditions or side effects and never really healing, then read on.

- *Genetics*: People ask me, "What about genetics? Why do some people smoke their whole lives and don't get lung cancer and somebody else gets a whiff of secondhand smoke and dies from cancer?" That's a great question, and here is the answer. All people have genetically strong areas in their bodies and areas that may be predisposed to certain conditions. Sometimes we learn of these areas through testing, and sometimes we never learn what they are until we develop an illness or disease of some sort. The point is that we all have an area that we could call our weakest link. Once enough toxins have been ingested, enough negative thoughts and emotions have been created, and enough stress has been created in our minds, our weakest link will begin to break down. So did the person who smoked his whole life and lived to eighty have superior lungs and heart?

Possibly, but what is more possible is that this person had superior thoughts each day. I am not suggesting that we can do whatever we want to our bodies and our minds will take care of it; again, our bodies have requirements. I will make a bold statement here. If you're watching the news every day, driving in traffic to a job you don't like, eating nonorganic food, and bathing in and drinking tap water, you will become ill if you have not already. The stress, the toxins, and the lack of proper nutrition together will send you to the doctor. Then once people begin to see a doctor, they generally continue to see the doctor because health care is not set up to make you healthy. The doctor is not skilled or trained to treat the causes of your illness, only the effects, which never cures anything.

So What Can We Do Then?

The next chapter lays out the guidelines for getting well and staying well. Remember to see a natural health practitioner for specific healing remedies and techniques. That being said, the following information is a baseline of things to do that have been proven to bring health back.

- First, realize that you have to be your own best doctor. Doctors certainly have their place, and I am not advocating that people not get routine checkups. Imaging today is so advanced that problem areas can be spotted and lives can be saved. That being said, it is up to you to do the right things each day so you can get or stay healthy. Be the doctor of prevention. Those same things that prevent disease can also reverse disease.

- Where are the three places disease and illness come from? What causes us to become acidic? Remember we talked about the fact that we don't catch diseases like cancer, diabetes, or heart disease out of the air like a germ or a virus. These major and widespread illnesses as well as countless others are conditions that we develop over time. Getting to the causes rather than just dealing with the effects—that is true health care.

Chapter 9

A Spiral Upward—
Addressing the Big Three

*H*ere are the *big* three causes of diseases that we will talk more about. The *big* three are as follows:

1. *Toxins*: We live in a toxic society.
2. *Proper Nutrition*: Organic is not enough.
3. *Poor Thinking and Negative Emotions*: Attitude is everything.

The big three, as I like to call them, affect our pH balance, which makes us acidic, which in turn negatively affects our health and ultimately causes illnesses to develop in our minds and bodies. Any one of the big three mentioned by itself can cause eventual breakdown of our health, leading to disease. Most people walking around are suffering from all three to some degree and are not even aware of it. Being susceptible to all three causes an exponential outcome on our health and becomes a matter of when, not if, an illness will show up.

Okay, now that we know the causes, let's look at how to remedy each of these issues. The information here is really an overview, and I encourage you to do your own research to discover more-detailed information on these topics. This information is not a secret. In fact, it is so simple that most people just don't realize how important it is. For the context of this book, we will be brief but also exact in our overviews.

All of the things I am going to share with you now are super powerful technologies and resources that have been around for a long time. If you have not heard of them or have heard negative press about any of them, just remember that the health care system does not make money by promoting health; the health care system deals with the aftermath of poor health. I am going to share with you ways to address the causes of illness and diseases, therefore bringing you back to health or preventing poor health in the first place. Do these things and your conditions will improve, whatever they are. I use or have used everything that follows, and thousands of others have used them, with outstanding results. Get happy because you are about to learn what the three issues are and how to get healthier and stay healthier. At first you may think there is simply too much to change here. But stay with me—you can get healthier and not be fanatical about it. Making one small change a week will put you in a completely different place health wise after a few months.

1. Toxins—from What and from Where?

The answer is they come from almost everything and everywhere. Toxins are accumulated in our bodies over time. Slowly toxins build up in our fat cells and major organs, including our brains. Our bodies are living sponges that absorb everything they come in contact with, good or bad. The problem is that society has led us to believe that many of the things that appear to be good on the surface are actually detrimental to our health. The fact is that 99 percent of the goods and services we consume each day are produced by companies that have no concern for our health. The companies are concerned with making money, and consumer beware is the policy. Before we can make changes, it is important to know what we need to change and why. Unless you live in a very remote place like Namibia or Galapagos, you are being bombarded with toxins by every aspect of modern-day living.

Let's look at some of the major areas where we are absorbing health-threatening toxins every day. We live in a toxic society. Therefore your first priority should be to remove the toxins or extremely reduce the toxins from your body and your lifestyle. You must get the toxins out! This is done through cleanses.

The first four cleanses I would recommend are, in this order: a colon cleanse, a fat-cell cleanse, a kidney-gallbladder cleanse, and a heavy metal cleanse. You can find many good cleansing products online or at your local health food store. The absolute best fat-cell cleanse on earth is something called the Purif at the Church of Scientology. This is also available elsewhere but may be a bit different at other facilities. I am not a Scientologist and neither do you need to be a Scientologist to go through this cleanse program. Read L. Ron Hubbard's book *Clear Body, Clear Mind* to understand why this one is so powerful. I was there for three weeks getting out the toxins. When I left, all of my senses were heightened because the toxins were gone. I could see better, food tasted better, and my mind was clearer. It is truly an amazing experience if you can do it. When my son (eighteen years old at the time) saw the changes that occurred in me, he wanted to go as well, so I sent him in for the treatment and he loved it.

There are other fat-cell cleanses you can do at home, of course. I'm just letting you know what is available to you. Remember, your brain is mostly fat, which is why the fat-cell cleanse is so important. A clear mind gives you a better outlook and attitude, as well as better problem-solving skills. It's huge.

Once you have gone through some cleansing, pick up silica, spirulina, and chlorella. This formula will keep you cleaned out and help keep you alkalized. Taking these three together three times a day is so powerful and does so many good things for your body. We will talk in more detail about this later. Do your own research, but if you are taking prescription or nonprescription drugs, form a plan to stop taking them with the help and support of your medical doctor. Consult your doctor and your natural health practitioner to work out a withdrawal plan. Just know that all drugs cause acidity in our bodies, and acidity is our enemy. Prescription and nonprescription drugs are poisons, make no mistake about it. I knew a young, beautiful, healthy teacher named Stacy who watched my kids when they were little. She died from an accidental overdose of acetaminophen—Tylenol. Stacy's kidneys shut down in response to the over-the-counter drug. This happens all the time but is not reported in the news. My doctor, who I had known and trusted for years, told me that I would need to take three drugs for the rest of my life. Guess what? I'm fifty-three and in perfect health now and do not take drugs to stay healthy. I took control of my health, and you can too.

Next, unless you are eating organic food, you are ingesting toxins. There's no way around it. The food in your favorite restaurant has toxins. Look at the table. See the sugar substitutes and the ketchup? Read the labels. High fructose corn syrup and the multiple chemicals in sugar substitutes cause so many health problems, from memory loss to cancer, that I cannot list them all in this tiny book. Buy organic food, and seek out organic restaurants. They are out there. Watch how much better you look and feel after a short time. Do the best you can to make these changes; you don't have to be a fanatic. It's a process that is well worth it, however long it takes to make these adjustments. Remember that toxins make your body more acidic, and when you're acidic, you are susceptible to disease setting in. Disease does not like an alkaline state or a pH-balanced body. Dr. Morter of Morter Health Systems, the man who really got me started on the path to health, stated, "Disease cannot exist in a pH-balanced body." Your doctor is not ever going to check your pH, so get some test strips online or at the local store and test yourself. Once you see that you are in fact acidic, making these changes should become easier for you.

We need to talk about water also when we are discussing toxins. Most tap water has all types of chemicals in it. If you are drinking it and bathing in it, you need to make changes. Buy a shower and water faucet filter from Fred Van Liew at ewaterdeal.com. These filters are the best I know of for taking out chlorine, fluoride, and other contaminants. As for bottled water, the best, cleanest, most naturally pH-balanced water is FIJI Water. Smartwater and most others are acidic with low vibration.

Last on the topic of removing or reducing intake of toxins is cosmetics, shampoos, soaps, lotions, and anything else skin bound. Here's a simple rule: if you can't ingest it, you don't want to put it on your body either. If your cosmetics, shampoos, toothpastes, lotions, etc., are not organic, they are toxic to you. Your local health food store has alternatives to these items, and if not, just go online to get what you need. Remember, your skin really is the largest organ on your body. What you absorb through it has an effect on your health. Just remember that toxins make you acidic, and being acidic allows illness and disease to set in. An acidic body is a body that is deteriorating. Get your body alkalized and you will stay healthier all of your life.

2. Proper Nutrition

The Greek physician Hippocrates proclaimed nearly twenty-five hundred years ago, "Let food be thy medicine and medicine be thy food." When Hippocrates was quoted as saying that, he wasn't talking about manmade, packaged, genetically modified, chemically enriched, acidity-causing food that lines the shelves of all major supermarkets today. Hippocrates was talking about eating food as close as possible to the way nature intended it. In countries where there has been famine or lack of quality food, people have disease. The body can go for a while without nutrition but then major organs begin to rob the rest of the body of minerals in order to keep a person alive until finally organs fail or the body develops a life threatening disease.

We don't need to be experts in nutrition, but we all need to know some basics. We also don't need to change everything we are doing all at the same time. Small changes, one by one, will put you on the path to health. For example, there is a reason why they say, "An apple a day keeps the doctor away." Everyone can eat one apple a day, and that small change does all kinds of great things for your health. One apple a day gives you flavonoids that fight diseases of the heart and cancer. Apples clean out your digestive tract, alkalizes the body, provides vitamin C and are delicious. How hard is it to grab an apple on the go? Today, however, you may want to grab a couple of apples a day. Can you grab some almonds on the go? Almonds are hugely alkalizing, have protein and minerals, and can lower cholesterol and fight colon cancer.

How hard is it to grab some delicious almonds rather that some silly peanuts, chips, or pretzels that cause you to be acidic? People need to eat more raw food, meaning food that hasn't had all of the nutrients cooked out of it. First, just know that on average, produce today in the United States is about five times less nutritious than it was fifty years ago. Then people cook their vegetables so they have almost no nutrition and add butter, salt, and pepper until it causes them to be acidic. Does this mean you can never have a hot meal? Of course not. Does this mean we need to eat five times the amount of food so we can get our nutrition? No, you just cannot eat enough food in a day to get all of the vitamins and minerals you need. It is simply a matter of learning what to eat and keeping in mind that your food should be as close as possible to the way nature intended it to be.

In addition, we will talk about supplementation. When I say supplementation, I don't mean vitamins and minerals tablets from the store. Those products do almost nothing for your health and have additives that actually hurt your health. Forget vitamins and mineral pills. If you want to turn your health around, just know that you need to eat more raw produce, less or no beef (unless it's organic, grass-fed beef), and nutritional supplements called whole food supplements or super foods. Whole food supplements are actual food that has complete nutrition. Super foods are not grown on US farms like produce.

Lack of proper nutrition invites disease all over the world. If you aren't taking a high-quality supplement, either whole food or liquid or powder, you simply have nutritional deficiencies. There's no way around it. Organic food is good because it is not genetically modified and doesn't have toxins in it. The bad news is that the nutritional content even in organic food is so far depleted now for a variety of reasons that you simply cannot eat enough food in a day to get the required minimums for optimal health. The good news is that you can eat almost anything you want, but eat food that is as close to nature intended if at all possible: raw apples, carrots, and spinach salad. As a rule, just know that if the food is not organic, it has toxins in it. This is the way it is today. Eat wild fish, not farm-raised fish. Most restaurant salmon and all tilapia is farm raised and hugely toxic. American beef that comes from corn-fed cows is destroying people's health. The cows are fed genetically modified corn feed with growth hormones and antibiotics. The cows are slaughtered in such a way that all of those toxins stay in the beef, which people then eat and take in those toxins. Eat beef only from grass-fed cows and chicken that is free range. Do a Google search to find the level of alkalinity versus acidity that different foods contain. You're going to want to eat 80 percent alkaline food or more in order to overcome an acidic condition.

Here are some (not all) of the most-alkaline foods (not counting super foods). In no particular order, you can find all of these at your supermarket, but always try to get organic: lemons (lemons were thought to be acidic but in fact the body converts it to alkaline quite nicely), lentils, green tea, fresh-squeezed juice, raw dates, grapefruit, grapes, limes, kiwis, papayas, mangos, pineapple, plums, raisins, tangerines, asparagus, onions, apple cider, sweet apples, alfalfa sprouts, apricots, ripe bananas, avocados, figs, nectarines, oranges, peaches, pears, almonds (not peanuts), raw chestnuts, sea salt, peaches, raspberries, beets, bell peppers, broccoli, cabbage, carrots, celery, sweet corn, garlic, fresh green beans, sweet peas, potato skin, kale, spinach, squash, sweet potatoes, and turnips.

Be Thankful

Be thankful for the food you eat. Thoughts are physical energy, and when focused, they can alter matter. That is proven science, not hocus pocus nonsense, watch the movie "What the bleep do we know". When you beam your appreciation at others, you are sending them good energy. It is the same with food. Some people pray before eating a meal. This spirit of appreciation actually puts good energy into the food just before you eat it. Food that is prepared with love is better for you from a vibration standpoint. A spirit of thankfulness alkalizes your body and puts your body in the correct state for optimally digesting the food and getting the most benefits from it. We will talk more about energy in the last and most important chapter, but know that being in a state of thankfulness allows your body to absorb nutrition.

When your body is at ease, it operates better. Disease is the opposite of being at ease. Find something to be thankful about, even when you are not eating throughout the day, even the smallest thing. You will know if you are being thankful because of the way you feel. Feeling good means you are being thankful. Do not eat when you are angry or upset. Go take a walk for thirty minutes and look out at the trees to relieve your negative energy. Walking is underrated and has huge health benefits. You want your body in a calm state when you eat. When you are stressed, you can feel your food getting hung up in your digestive tract. This causes issues such as acid reflux and constipation. When your food backs up and doesn't flow, you begin to have all kinds of health issues. Toxins need to be released and flow out of you easily, so make your eating time a time of calmness, and share that time only with others who share this attitude.

Going back to supplementation, we have to talk a little about juicing. Juicing is not quite as convenient as other supplements but is one of the best ways to get your whole food nutrition. I recommend buying a juicing book so when you do it for the first time, you actually put fruits and veggies in a proper recipe. Some people throw some random fruits or veggies in a juicer, and then when they drink it, it doesn't taste good so they stop. Although it may be healthy, if it doesn't taste good, people won't consume it. A juicing book can show you ways to put produce together so it not only tastes good but will also maximize the benefits. People juice to cleanse, to lose weight, to gain energy, to normalize blood pressure, and for many other benefits. Again, let's keep in mind that if you are acidic (which can be checked with test strips), you want to eat about 80 percent alkaline foods. As I mentioned earlier, you can find charts online that show some of the most-alkaline to most-acidic foods.

Mixing Proteins and Starches

This one is hugely important for health and can be implemented right now, and you won't have to purchase anything you don't already have. In life there are many examples of say a recipe or a formula in which the ingredients or the individual components work together to create an exponential effect. If a component is left out or a wrong component is added to the proven recipe or formula, you do not get the optimal results, if any results. So it is with eating. Some foods work well together, and some do not.

Without giving you a ton to think about, we can make this very easy. Proteins require acid in the stomach to break down in the digestive process. Carbohydrates or (starches) require alkaline to be broken down in the digestive process. Acid and alkaline are both needed for a balanced pH. However, when we eat proteins (meat, fish, poultry) and carbs or starches (bread, rice, potatoes) together, our digestion process slows way down, causing food to sit and rot in our stomachs, which in turn causes many health issues, the least of which are stomachaches, acid reflux, bloating, constipation, etc. This is because the acid that is attempting to break down the protein is being counteracted by the alkaline that is breaking down the carbs or starches. The proteins and the carbs together basically cause the body to continue to work hard by supplying more acid to the protein until finally the food goes down, leaving you fatigued and not feeling great.

The solution is to eat your proteins with greens or other vegetables and carbs or starches by themselves. This one change will help your health because your digestive tract won't keep food and waste in your body. People generally don't realize how important proper digestion of food is. What you don't digest properly doesn't help you and what you don't expel properly can hurt you. This is why raw fruits and vegetables are so important. It is not only for nutrition but just as important fruits and veggies support and enable proper digestion and elimination.

The Amazing Three-Food Formula for Supreme Health!

For our last section on the topic of nutrition, let's talk more specifically about something I mentioned earlier in the book. I recommend that you incorporate the following things into your daily diet, and when you do, they will have profound effects on your health. If you do nothing else, take the following information and try it for sixty days, and watch what happens to your skin, your hair, your energy levels, and most of all, the way you feel. Do you want your blood pressure to be 120/80 like mine and have no illnesses or chronic conditions?

It is easy, and you will be amazed. There are three components to the formula, each component having superior benefits to your health. When we combine all three together, the benefits are exponential. The formula was given to me by a very spiritual friend of mine named Alfred who received it from a person who channeled the formula. I encourage you to do a little research online so you can see for yourself how powerful each component is for the human body. When all three are taken together, they do all of the right things to send your ailments away and give you vibrant health.

Enter Spirulina

The first component is spirulina. Spirulina or (blue-green algae) is very alkalizing to the body, but it has many, many other benefits to your health. Entire books have been written on spirulina, but we will hit a few of the highlights here. Spirulina is considered to be a complete food in and of itself. Spirulina that comes from the bottom of deep freshwater lakes has highly concentrated phytonutrients and high amounts of chlorophyll, which simply is not contained in the greens you buy at the produce stand. The combination of amino acids, proteins, B complex vitamins, beta carotene, complex carbs, and iron gives the body superior nutrition.

The high-antioxidant value alone serves the body and protects the cells. People take spirulina for better digestion because it promotes good bacteria growth and flora, which allows better nutrition absorption and healthy bowel functions.

People use spirulina to clean the body of toxins, including heavy metals. People take it to strengthen the immune system and lower blood pressure. People take it for brain and liver protection. Taking this one-food supplement alone will increase the overall health of a body and help to keep the body from becoming acidic. I will share how to take this supplement at the end of this section.[1]

Enter Chlorella

The second component is called chlorella. Like spirulina, chlorella is very alkalizing. Chlorella is a powerful detoxifier. It is especially effective at removing heavy metals from the body. Metals like cadmium, mercury, and lead, which accumulate in the body, cause all kinds of health issues in the brain, and chlorella works at getting them out. Chlorella is such a good cleanser of the body that many believe that it fights arthritis, cancer, and other degenerative diseases. Chlorella is believed to normalize blood sugar and blood pressure. Chlorella has vitamins such as E, B, and C as well as zinc. Chlorella is rich in magnesium, which in itself performs hundreds of beneficial processes in the body.

---

[1]   Blinkova LP, Gorobets OB, Baturo AP. Biological activity of Spirulina. *Zh Mikrobiol Epidemiol Immunobiol.* 2001;(2): 114–18.

Chlorella strengthens the immune system, which means prevention from and faster healing of injury, illness, and disease. Always remember these claims are not supported by the FDA. Like spirulina, chlorella is a super food, and health claims have been documented by the many people who take it. I will share how to take this supplement in the end of this section.[2]

Enter Silica

The third and last component is silica. Silica isn't talked about a whole lot. Our food, however, has been depleted of this very important compound, and it is vital for our overall health. Silica is a trace element that is crucial to overall physical health. It is water soluble and therefore needs to be refreshed in the body daily. The health of our connective tissues and collagen relies on a steady source of silica. Silica strengthens our joint tissues, ligaments, and muscles. It is what keeps our skin from sagging on the outside and heart muscles working well on the inside. Silica promotes calcium absorption, which keeps bones strong. A deficiency in silica causes people to look and feel older than their years. Plenty of silica in our diet promotes new cell growth and can be seen through healthier hair and skin, as well as fingernail and toenail growth.

---

[2]   Dhyana Bewicke and Beverly A. Potter, *Chlorella, the Emerald Food.* (Berkeley, CA: Ronin Publishing Inc., 1984); Dr. David Steenbock, *Chlorella Natural Medicine Algae.* (Mission Viejo, CA: Aging Research Institute, 1996); Paul Pitchford, *Healing with Whole Foods, Third Edition.* (Berkeley, CA: North Atlantic Books, 2002).

I can tell you after my first few weeks of silica supplementation, I saw improvements in my skin, small wrinkles disappeared, my hair got softer and healthier, and my fingernails and toenails got stronger. When I went to visit my mother a few months ago, she said, "Kurt you're the best I've ever seen you." Now I'm fifty-three, not twenty-three, so when she said that I knew something was working. Sometimes when we can actually see results with our eyes, they become more real, but just think of what is going on inside of the body as well. There are many more benefits to silica supplementation. Do your own research.

I will share the best form of silica out there to take, which has even more benefits than just plain silica, such as removing parasites from the digestive tract. I will also share how best to take the supplement at the end of this section.

Taking the Three-Food Formula

All three of the components above can be purchased at your local health food store or online, and when all three are taken together, they have an exponential effect on your health. Here is how I recommend taking them.

- I take the spirulina in capsule/powder form, although you may take it in liquid or powder form as well. Read the label to understand what one serving is. For detoxification on the first week, take one serving a day. In the second week, take two servings a day. In the third week, take three servings a day. Stay at three servings a day for ninety days, and then you can go back down to a serving a day (maintenance serving) for as long as you would like to stay in supreme health. For longer detox requirements, you can keep up the three servings a day for a year if you like. Remember, it is food.

- I take the chlorella (from Japan) in compressed tablet form, although you may take it in liquid or powder form as well. Read the label to understand what one serving is. For detoxification in the first week, take one serving a day. In the second week, take two servings a day. In the third week, take three servings a day. Stay at three servings a day for ninety days, and then you can go back down to a serving a day (maintenance serving) for as long as you would like to stay in supreme health. For longer detox requirements, you can keep up the three servings a day for a year if you like. Remember, it is food.

- I take the silica in a different form than a standard silica supplement. Now you can certainly buy silica in capsule or liquid form, but here is the best way to buy and take your silica. Some local health stores have it, but I buy online. It is called diatomaceous earth food grade, and it is about 80 percent silica and has added benefits to the silica you are taking. Do a little research on what a diatom is. Diatoms run through your entire body, cleaning it of residue and toxins. The tiny diatoms' sharp edges cut and remove parasites hiding out in the digestive tract and also clean our arteries of buildup caused by being acidic. The silica is excellent, and the added benefits of having little bottle brushes cleaning you out is fantastic for your overall health.

Take all three of the above together each day. I take my first servings the very first thing in the morning before anything else. If you do this first thing in the morning, you will gain energy, and the formula goes right to work on your body, which hasn't had food or water for eight hours.

Please note: Because people are so loaded up with toxins, sometimes when people start a cleansing regime like this, they think they are experiencing side effects and feel bad in the beginning. In reality, they are experiencing the effects of detoxification. The cleansing process has broken loose toxins, and the body is in the process of trying to eliminate them. You may get gas, nausea, stomach cramps, diarrhea, etc. This is good! It means it's working. Stay with it, though, and once a lot of the loose toxins have been eliminated, you will start to feel better and better. Drink lots and lots of clean purified water during this time and you will be fine.

3. Poor Thinking and Negative Emotions—Attitude Is Everything

This is the last of the big three and probably the most important. We must get our thinking right in order to be healthy and happy. Many people do not understand that your mind is the most powerful medicine you have access to. Negative thinking causes negative emotions like fear, worry, doubt, anger, frustration, and depression. These emotions wear on your body and cause your body to become acidic, which invites disease. Positive thinking, on the other hand, causes good-feeling emotions such as optimism, appreciation, hopefulness, enthusiasm, love, contentment, and laughter, which alkalize your body, therefore strengthening your immune system as well as all bodily functions.

Many people don't realize just how negative their overall thinking is and has been. It takes a conscious effort to change the patterns of our thinking due to the neuro pathways that have been developed in the brain over the years, but it can and must be done. It is easy to know if your thinking is negative or positive; just check your emotions. Your good-feeling emotions tell you if your attitude is correct. Your bad-feeling emotions tell you that your thinking is incorrect and in need of change. Keeping your mind focused on the result you want and not the problem is the single most important thing you can do when you have an illness. Most people who are ill, however, may say, "Well, of course I want to get well," yet they continue to focus on the illness and not wellness. Does that make sense to you? If you continue to focus on what is, you will continue to get what is. You must focus on what you want and not on what you don't want. Whatever you focus on (whether you want it or not) you will get more of it. This is science, not hocus pocus. Your brain does not understand, "I don't want this illness" Your brain just hears "illness." Even Captain Jack Sparrow from the movie *Pirates of the Caribbean* got it right when he said, "The problem is not the problem. The problem is your attitude about the problem."

There is so much scientific data now to support the fact that your mind controls every aspect of your body. It is not up for debate any longer. There are hundreds of documented cases of people getting well simply because they believed they could and focused on that result while feeling good about it. The best time to get your thinking right is before you become ill, but of course you can still turn yourself around if you are ill. Most of us don't realize that our good health is our single most precious resource until it has been taken from us.

Reading some good, uplifting material every day is vital. When I read and learn something positive first thing in the morning, I can't help but feel better, and that sets the tone for the entire day with a smile.

Don't watch the news. The media instills fear and worry into your mind. It's not news; it's drama and distraction there to make us feel less than good. The same goes for mainstream media in general. It's not there to make you feel good. Advertising in general attempts to and does get into your mind. Guard your mind, and only allow good information to enter. Your mind controls your body. Feed your mind constantly with good information and good thoughts. You may need to consider new friends or looking for groups of like-minded individuals. Meet-up groups are great for this and are free or very cheap to attend. I created a meet-up group here in Clearwater. We have over one hundred people of like minds, and we talk about all of this information on a regular basis. I watch people's lives change right before my eyes. Making these changes *will* change your life. Some people think, *I thought there would be some sort of secrets or magic in this book,* but the truth is that these basics are the magic.

The fact is that our mind controls every aspect of our bodies. If we are not at ease in our minds, we cause disease in our bodies. So yes, we want to give good nutrition, exercise, and rest to our bodies. These are requirements. Gas and oil and tires are requirements for a car to run correctly, but if I get in the car and drive it off a cliff, that nice car is ravaged or destroyed. It is the same with our day-to-day thoughts and the effects those thoughts have on our bodies.

Our goal as people, whether we are ill or not, is to always try to feel a little better. We can't always be feeling blissful, but we can always try to feel a little better. There are many ways to do this. When we look for something to appreciate, we feel better. All people have something they can appreciate. Being thankful and appreciating what we do have puts us in the correct state for healing—that alkalizing state. Books like *The Magic of Believing*, *The Power of Positive Thinking*, and *The Anatomy of an Illness* are must reads if you are ill. These books are stories of real people with real issues who overcome those issues and get what they want through the power of their thoughts. When you read these types of books, you begin to say, "Hey, if he or she did it, so can I."

We all need to be purposely putting good mental nutrition into our brains every day just as we put nutrition into our bodies. Do this through the use of good books, good audiobooks and the company of good-quality, uplifting people. We cannot sit and watch the news every day and expect to feel good. Without getting all sinister about it, as I said earlier, the media is not there to make you feel good. It instills fear and promotes agendas and is generally talking about things that have no relevance to your life. Occasionally when I am at a hotel, I will turn on the news just to check in. They are still talking about the same issues. It's about different people and different places but the same old story, and none of it is useful. You want to feel better? Turn off the TV and open a book. Get audiobooks. They are great. You can learn so much through audiobooks while driving or doing other things around the house.

Chapter 10

Changing Your Thoughts, Changing Your Life

*N*ow, I know a lot of you are saying, "Yeah, I've heard all of this stuff before. I know, I know."

Well, remember what Leo Buscaglia said: "To know and not to do is really not to know."

In other words, if you aren't doing it, then you may as well not know about it. Not all people are in the same place with this material. Some people believe the mind-body connection, and some are struggling with the concepts because of the heavy programming done by the media and society. That programming in general has been done to sell you something.

One of the most powerful discoveries that proves people can think their way into recovery that has been proven over and over again is the placebo effect. The placebo effect is simply where patients are given a worthless treatment, drug (sugar pill), or procedure but told that it will cure them. In many studies, it is documented that 30 to 40 percent of those patients became well again purely because they thought they were being given something that would heal them. Could there be any better evidence?

What these studies don't report and I would like to add is this: If we could have gotten the remainder of the group's thinking correct—gotten them to truly believe they would be well again—that 30 to 40 percent number would be much higher. Most Americans underestimate the power of one's thoughts, faith, and beliefs. Americans have been conditioned to believe that the power lies somewhere else other than inside of each one of us. Think about it—the reason the placebo works is because of the belief in the doctor that gave it to the patients. Those doctors, however, did nothing and have no magical powers. The healing came from the people themselves, not from another person or a substance.

People talk about miracles. What is a miracle? Well, in the Bible, a blind man came to Jesus and asked for healing. Jesus replied, "What do you want me to do for you?"

The blind man said, "I want to regain my sight."

Jesus said to him, "Go. Your faith has made you well."

The man immediately regained his sight. Was that a miracle, or could it be high belief that causes what are considered to be miracles? Some people I know say, "Well, I'll believe it when I see it." Guess what? They never see it! What you believe to be true is what you see, and a belief is nothing more than thoughts that have been thought over and over again.

The good news is that you can change your thoughts and beliefs in one second, and that is the basis for bringing on a miracle. Miracles do not happen to non-believers.

Do you still doubt that your thoughts or your psychological states can affect the body's biology, for better or worse? It is documented that some people with multiple personality disorders also have multiple physiologies. What does that mean? Here's an example of one I read about. Here is a guy named Bob. Bob has diabetes. Bob also has another personality in which he is David. Remember, having multiple personalities is a purely psychological illness. Bob has been diagnosed with diabetes for a long time. David, the alter personality, does not have diabetes. When Bob is provoked to become David, the diabetes is gone! When they test Bob's blood, he has diabetes, but a few minutes later when they test Bob's blood again while in his altered personality state of David, there is no sign of diabetes. This is evidence of the mind altering the physiology of the body. Now I am not advocating that you develop a second personality in order to cure an illness; I am simply giving examples of how the power of one's beliefs brings manifestations to our physical bodies as well as our life in general. When we focus more on wellness than illness, the balance will shift to wellness. Where your attention goes, energy flows.

You cannot make something unwanted go away by thinking about it. You must think about what you want, not what you don't want, in order to make the shift. Henry Ford said, "If you think you can or you think you can't, either way you're right. It's the thinking that makes it so." These little quotes that I have included throughout the book are not just cute phrases. There is science behind each one of them. Work on your mind, protect your mind from negative influences, and use your power of thought to make the changes you want to see.

Chapter 11

Go for Your Dreams

A final statement and probably the most powerful concept of this short book is this: if there is one thing you can do in order to think better thoughts, feel better emotions, have better health, and have a truly happy, rewarding life, it is to go for your dreams. The happiest, healthiest people are those who are creating and manifesting their dreams. When we humans are in the process of creating something we want in our lives, it does all of the right things for us.

I believe we are creative beings here to create and cocreate. How do I know this? Because when we are creating, going after a goal or a dream or a desire, we feel good! And when we feel good emotionally, our bodies do the right thing. We are alkalized, energized, and passionate. That is our true nature.

When we were kids, everything was exciting and amazing and unfolding before our eyes. Anything was possible. When you are thinking about or doing something you love, everything else takes care of itself like magic. It can be as small as ordering a book online and getting excited to read it. It can be making plans to go to Hawaii and watching the calendar for the time to come. Write that book, learn to play that instrument, or do whatever you can from where you are right now that will make you feel a little better. Just take the first step. People become stuck when they ask themselves, "How will I be able to do this? How will I be able to do that? What if this happens, or what if that happens?" Forget about how and think about why you're going to be, do, or have something you want. The why is where your power is. The how will show up when you have enough why energy behind it. Reread that last sentence because that is powerful. We can't wait for the world to change around us; we must make the changes. Gandhi said, "Be the change you want to see in the world."

I believe what he meant by that is that when we change, what we see in our world changes. Make just small changes and you will see big results. Then you will want to make more changes and then more. You don't have to change everything all at once and you don't need all of the answers, but do get started. Zig Zigglar said, "Go as far as you can see. Then when you get there, you'll see a little further." Just take one step, such as going through one cleanse. There is power and momentum in that first step. Once you do that and see how good you feel, you may want to do another cleanse and another. There really is no right or wrong order. Everyone is different, and it's not a race. You may decide to eat an apple a day or take a walk each evening. These are small but powerful changes, and one successful change will inspire another, then another change. Go get the spirulina, chlorella, and silica formula and see what happens to your overall health. Take that first step for your health and your life.

Kevin Trudeau, who taught me so much about health and life, said success is a decision away. This means that all of your power to change your health or anything else will come from you making a decision. Make a decision that no matter what has to be done to get healthy, you will do it and you will take responsibility. You must finally get sick and tired of being sick and tired (literally). You must take 100 percent responsibility for your health and not blame the doctors, your heredity, or your upbringing. Make the decision to be healthy, and know that you will be healthy. Picture in your mind your vision of how you will look and what you will be doing once you have regained your health. Stop thinking of the illness, and start thinking about wellness. Your mind is the most powerful tool you have to regain and keep your health. Knowing that, turn off the TV and the bad news. Keep reading inspirational books, and spend time with encouraging people.

I hope this information was helpful in your journey to health and well-being.

Following the principles in this small book is all you need to begin to change your health for the better. Due to many requests, I have created a high quality pre-mixed 30-day supply of the Chlorella, Spirulina, Silica health formula described in the book. This gets people started in the right direction quickly. I also provide one on one and group coaching in the areas of stress reduction as well as mental, emotional and physical health.

Keep an eye out for future books and services that delve deeper into these principles. I look forward to serving you. For more information, simply write to me at: kwinowich@gmail.com

Be well, Kurt Winowich